Andy Baxter introduces you to Terri, Debby, Betty a at
become today's legends. This book has a digestible a
empowers people to health. He has the unique persp
many sides of fitness. He is an accomplished world cl
The Baxter Plan is encouraging, enthusiastic and pro.
though a short book, he focuses on the right words, at the right time, for the right situation
and an intention that will yield miraculous outcomes. These pages are peppered with stories
of everyday people attaining new heights. "Know this; your functional independence and
quality of life are depending on you to be powerful and to endure".

P. Michael Stone MD, MS, IFMCP
Faculty Institute for Functional Medicine
International educator, author, clinician in nutrition and functional Medicine

This book is an enjoyable, easy-reading, no-nonsense look at why moving our bodies is vital
to our health and quality of life. With a good sense of humor and real-life examples of people
changing their lives through exercise, Andy shows us how we can get the most out of exercise
and even make it fun! With this book, Andy joins fellow Personal Lifestyle Medicine
professionals around the world who are showing us how each of us as individuals can take
the future of our health, well-being, and functionality into our own hands.

Laura Robin, DO, MPH

Andy Baxter's latest book, *The Exercise Prescription* is a prescription for empowerment. I enjoyed
reading about his clients' personal stories and appreciate his entertaining writing style with the
clear message that exercise as we age (at every stage in life) is the foundation of well-being.

Julie K. Kokinakes, RDN, LDN
Medical Nutrition Therapist in private practice

So many facts and truths inside. Relating these truths to patients/clients is good.
Good job!

Jill Steinsiek, MD

Andy Baxter has developed a program for middle-age and senior people that combines sound
exercise principles with the aging body. Truly this is a masterful approach that tailors one's
program to fit any diagnosis. I have recommended his facilities to many patients. It really works!

Patrick Wedlake, DO

Andy's writing is delightful and captivating. More importantly, he debunks several exercise
fitness myths. Most importantly, he is inspiring both to those among his readers who need to
start on a path to functional fitness as well as those among his readers who need a boost to
continue on one. He offers sound and practical advice to both.

Cornelia Byers, MD
Fellow American Academy of Physical Medicine & Rehabilitation

THE EXERCISE
Prescription

ANDY BAXTER, MES, PRCS

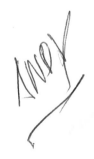

Acknowledgments

This book is dedicated to each and every one of my inspirational members.

Special thanks to Anna Elkins and Robert Frost for helping me put this little book together.

Forward

In life we discover great if we are fortunate. Rarely do we encounter brilliant mastery. Andy Baxter has demonstrated mastery with his elegantly simple and thoughtful work, The Exercise Prescription. Andy clearly demonstrates his philosophy that fitness is essential to a fulfilled life. This text will help you achieve fitness and motivate you to continue.

As a physician who has trained with some of the best in medicine at Stanford and UCLA, I am very impressed by the expertise and inspiration that Andy so skillfully presents in this timely text.

Thank you Andy!

John Delgado, MD

Table of Contents

INTRODUCTION: Why Am I Writing This Book?

I grew up in a fitness family. We were an active, outdoorsy bunch. I got my introduction to strength training as a kid from my cousin Ed. He worked at the North Berkeley, CA YMCA and did personal training out of his basement. He was already hooked on fitness, and he helped me become a lifelong student of it.

I ran cross-country in elementary school, found boxing in junior high, played soccer in high school, and rowed in college. As a master oarsman I had the good fortune to rack up well over a dozen US and Canadian National championships, two World Championships, and even got a chance to compete for a spot on the 2008 Olympic team. It was a great adventure and an even greater story, so I wrote a book about it, *Racing Yesterday*. I am currently a member of the very first USA men's master's raft team. We competed alongside 76 teams from 28 countries to win the Bronze medal at the 2016 world championships; also a grand adventure.

I started my first personal training business as a student at NYU. Now, 28 years later, there isn't much that I haven't seen or done in the fields of senior fitness, sports performance and medical exercise. I have worn the hats of athlete, author, coach, senior trainer, gym owner, medical exercise specialist, consultant, inventor, and worldwide public speaker at the junior-, master-, professional- and Olympic levels of athletics, the medical community, and the athletic equipment industry.

I tell you all of this because in my experiences and interactions with every walk of life within these varied disciplines, I am still educating on the same topics and answering the *same questions* over and over again, fighting the good fight against an ever–growing, self-perpetuating, $21.4 billion-dollar "fitness" industry. As it is with the food industry, it is increasingly difficult to delineate truth from cunning marketing rhetoric when it comes to exercise.

And so I wrote this book.

Sure, it's a little book. But just like exercise, it's the quality of the content, not the quantity. This slim little book is a powerhouse of strength. Less is more.

As you read, you'll find answers—real, truthful answers to recurring dogmas—to finally dispel and debunk the most prolific myths about exercise currently out there.

Exercise has profoundly beneficial applications, both as prevention and as treatment, for our bodies' integrated systems.

If you're reading this, I'm guessing you want to keep those systems in top working order. And I'm guessing you've asked doctors or personal trainers a question or two about how to do that. These answers are for you, and this book is my "prescription" for a life of fitness. May it educate, clarify, and empower you!

Sincerely,
Andy Baxter, MES, PRCS

CHAPTER 1: Attitude is Almost Everything

I own a gym called *Baxter Fitness Solutions for Fifty and Beyond*. In the course of any given day, my staff and I will see a broad range of folks. There are the perfectly healthy ones just looking for a good place to exercise. And then there are the ones in various states of disrepair—generally due to specific conditions related to aging and disuse. These people enter with existing ailments that can't be simply checked at the door: Parkinson's, multiple sclerosis, stroke, cancer, orthopedic conditions, brain trauma, metabolic disorders, and multiple combinations thereof.

Every one of these conditions has its own cruel symptoms: pain, fatigue, anxiety, physical limitation, depression, neurologic and speech limitations, functional shortcomings, etc. The list goes and on and on with subsets of each that go on and on….

Regardless of their symptoms, each person who makes their way through our door has one, fully functioning power over which they have complete control: *attitude*. Attitude is what shapes and defines our character. Attitude is more relevant than money, social standing, proprietary holding, or vanity. Attitude decimates the playing field and beats the pants off of our seeming limitations.

Ironically, a positive attitude can be found radiating from the eyes and smiles and hearts of those coping with terrible ailments. In the face of adversities, these people keep their positive attitudes, and they show up.

Here's a good example: I was visiting with my friend Virgil two days ago. Virgil made an appearance in my first book, *Racing Yesterday*. He's the Cal pitching ace who struck out Yale's George "Poppy" Bush to win the very first College World Series and turn pro with the Oakland Oaks. Virgil is 92 years old. As spry and witty as ever, he told me, "Exercise and attitude. That's all there really is, isn't there?"

That got me thinking; how many clients do I have over the age of 70? 80? 90?

Since I'm on a baseball bent, I decided to crunch the numbers, and they are inspiring. Of our devoted, active agers, 201 are in their 70s, 64 are in their 80s and 10 are in their 90s. These are people who are making the active decision to get off their butts, get out of their homes, get down to the gym and get active.

As I write this, Alma and Bill are working out, side by side. Like Virgil, Bill is 92. He and Alma have been married for 64 years. Now there's a great example of two people who know the power of showing up—and a positive attitude! In marital bliss stats, Bill is batting a lifetime average of .696. Ty Cobb, eat your heart out.

Showing up is everything. A positive attitude is a close second.

YOUR PRESCRIPTION:

This first one is pretty obvious: Get moving! Find something that makes you happy, that is compatible with who you are, that you look forward to, that becomes a routine part of your life. I have a friend who fenced in college. Then life happened. Long story short, after a successful professional career and raising two children, she rediscovered her passion for fencing, recently returning from Puerto Rico with three Golds and a Bronze at the Master Fencing Championships. It is a great fit for her. Maybe it's tango, or tennis, or swimming, or surfing—whatever it is, don't think of it as a chore or a punishment. Showing up is no small thing, so you should WANT to show up!

CHAPTER 2: Do Not Go Gentle

I have been working with aging athletes and adventurers for over twenty years. I work with people who have undertaken athletic challenges for the first time in their forties, fifties, and sixties, and I work with people who are still athletes and adventurers in their eighties and even in their nineties. As an athlete myself, I am concerned with maintaining my own ability to perform at the highest level. I am continuously amazed at how rapidly our understanding is changing about what is humanly possible at any given age.

In the last few years, however, I've been working to help people understand something more fundamental—something that separates the still potential athlete and adventurer from someone sliding headlong down a slippery slope. The ultimate dividing line is often what we call "the fall," that little slip that becomes catastrophic. But decades before that actual catastrophe takes place, an insidious process begins that might best be described as the "fear of falling." That fear gradually saps our strength and confidence— ultimately becoming a self-fulfilling prophecy.

Preventing falls takes effort, but mostly it requires understanding how the fear is set in motion. Most of all, we need to recognize that the first tremors of the fear of falling are a call to action: specifically a call to lift weights.

Anatomy of a Fall

Falls are typically a disastrous cocktail made of three compromised ingredients: strength, confidence, and range of motion (ROM).

Loss of Strength due to age-related muscle atrophy, called sarcopenia, reduces confidence and ROM.

Loss of Confidence due to injury and/or age reduces strength through muscle inhibition and reduces ROM.

Loss of ROM due to injury, associated atrophy, neurologic incident (stroke, Parkinson's, MS) reduces strength and confidence.

In other words, the source of the fall is not a sudden obstacle, a change in direction, or misjudging the height of the step. We deal successfully with that sort of situation throughout our lives. Instead, the source of the fall is weakness, fear, and limited

ROM that eventually creates the accident. The good news is that improving any one of these three factors has been shown to have a positive impact on the other two. Increasing your confidence will measurably increase your strength and ROM. Increasing your ROM will increase your strength and confidence. Increasing your strength is most important of all—and will most dramatically improve your confidence and ROM.

Why the Slope Gets Slippery

Before we take another step forward, I want to clear up some basic misconceptions about strength and aging that I encounter all the time. Muscle is muscle, fat is fat. Muscle does not turn into fat. Fat does not turn into muscle. Muscle is dense tissue, about 18 percent denser than fat. Muscle is also much more metabolically active than fat, so a fit body has a higher metabolism. As we age, we lose muscle—typically 4/10ths of one pound of muscle per year after 50. Less muscle means our metabolism slows, so we tend to gain weight. But even if our weight stays the same, our volume increases—which means we float better and our clothes no longer fit. What's more significant is that we have a larger body to support even as we have less strength to support it. Making matters worse is that our muscles are a major part of what's called our proprioceptive system that tells us where we are in space. As we age, we tend to become larger and less dense even as we get weaker and less in touch with where we are. It's the perfect set up for a fall.

"But I walk, I don't need anything else," is something I hear a lot—especially from practical people who design their dream homes without stairs. To me, it's almost as if they're in a hurry to qualify for one of those "free" scooters advertised on TV. Walking is great for your heart and your mood, but it's an inefficient form of exercise from a musculoskeletal perspective. I have many clients who can walk but who can't get out of a chair or rake leaves or pick up their grandchildren. They are not only missing out on life, they are heading for a fall. People should build their dream houses with plenty of stairs!

"So what is the best way to avoid a fall?", people finally ask. And that question gets to the primary goal of exercising the aging body from a musculoskeletal standpoint. What you want to do is to preserve functional strength, which is another way of saying you want to preserve muscle, confidence, and ROM. Assuming you are healthy and free from major medical deficits, you have a lot of fine and enjoyable choices to choose from, including Leki stick trail hiking, cross-country skiing, yoga, Pilates, martial arts, dance, rowing, horseback riding, swimming, and fencing. All of these types of exercise are great for ROM and confidence. Just keep in mind that the optimum health strategy includes one or more of these activities, plus a regular weight routine to specifically work on building and maintaining muscle.

The safest and most effective way to build muscle for older people is using resistance modalities that create compound (multi-joint), closed chain, non-concussive movements with optimal range of motion such that the muscles are supporting the skeleton and not the other way around. While all that sounds complicated, it's not really.

A compound movement involves two or more joints working together with their associated musculature. Imagine a rowing movement with the upper body. In that movement both your elbows and shoulder joints are moving together, so you are sharing the load between the two sets of joints. To accomplish this move you are firing the muscles of the forearms, upper arms, posterior shoulders, upper back, and middle back. No need to name all of the muscles exactly, just know that there is a lot going on in a compound movement. Typically, compound movements are closed chain, which essentially means the hands or feet are in contact with either the ground or with a machine. That stability increases safety.

Aerobic examples of great compound movements are cycling (either recumbent or upright, depending on ability and/or need for spinal support), rowing, upper body ergometers, and recumbent steppers. Strength examples would be squats, leg presses, seated rows, dead lifts, and high pulls. With all these movements good form is critical. Consult with a qualified trainer so that you can properly ingrain the right patterns into your neuromuscular memory. Once you have established the proper pattern, the rest is comparatively easy!

Less effective and potentially more dangerous weight exercises are open chain, primary rotary movements, such as leg curls, dumbbell "flyes," and hip adduction/abduction machines. Adding weight to the end of our lever arm or leg puts a lot of more stress (the bad kind) on our working parts than compound movements. While such movements can be very helpful in some circumstances (including injury rehabilitation), you don't want to do them without a clear purpose and supervision.

Things like stomach crunches and hip abduction/adduction machines are what we loosely call vanity movements: inefficient, ineffective, and potentially injurious. Save your open chain movements for the therapeutic environment where joint stability and range of motion are the order of the day. Focus instead on big, functional, compound movements that will keep you strong, loose, and not afraid to do the things you love.

YOUR PRESCRIPTION:

What if you could progress faster by peddling backward? Sure, you know how to pedal a bike smoothly and evenly and fluidly; you learned as a kid and have reinforced that neuromuscular pattern through millions of revolutions. But try pedaling backwards under a similar load with those same dynamic qualities and, at least initially, you will look and feel like a klutz; the movement will be jerky and the pressure uneven—like brushing your teeth with your opposite hand. Why? Because these new movements are foreign to your dominant neuromuscular hardwiring. Introducing new and varied neuromuscular patterning improves kinesthesia, proprioception, and motor skills for fall prevention, and that's just the short list. The field of neuroplasticity and neurogenesis is burgeoning and the evidence in support of safe and effective exercise is irrefutable. In other words, Just do it…*differently!*

CHAPTER 3: Breaking the Cycle of Fear

The patient says to the doctor: "Doc, it hurts when I do this" So the doctor nods her head sagely and replies, "Don't do that."

You've probably heard that one before. Well, funny or not, there is a flaw in that medical advice. As a medical exercise specialist, I see the pain/fear avoidance model walk through my door just about every day in one form or another. Let me explain. When it comes to movement and exercise, we have three typical responses to pain.

One: We fear the pain, so we avoid the activity that causes the pain—and we ultimately sink into disability and depression.

Two: We mask the pain with pills and shots, so we create unnecessary damage—and we ultimately sink into disability and depression.

Three: We do not fear the pain, so we are able listen to it and figure out exactly what it is telling us to do next—and we recover and get on with our active lives.

For example: A few years ago, Betty developed what she self-diagnosed as severe hip pain. It hurt when she did certain activities, so she stopped doing them. Then she tried doing other activities, but they hurt too, so she stopped doing them as well. Then she just stopped.

Fast forward—actually *slow, painful* forward—three years. Betty is now in constant pain and much heavier than when the pain started. When she comes to my fitness center, we discover that her hip pain is not actually hip pain at all. Hip pain typically presents itself in one of three ways: in the butt and low back (posterior), on the side (lateral), or in the front (anterior). Anterior hip pain is referred to as "true" hip pain. Betty's pain is presenting on the side; her foot is turned out (rotated externally) and her knee is caved in toward her midline (valgus collapse). What that means is that Betty is actually suffering from a wicked—and common—case of IT Band Friction Syndrome. When the iliotibial band (a stubborn strip of fascia that runs from the ilium down the side of the leg to the tibia on the outside of the knee) is overly tight or aggravated, it pulls structures out of alignment, inhibits muscle function, and *hurts like hell.*

I explain all this to Betty. Then, with Betty seated on medically specialized exercise machines, I cue her to rotate her foot into a vertical position. This makes her knee cave in more, so we identify that. She then makes the conscious decision to align her knee directly over her foot. As she goes through her various exercises and activities, she is vigilant to maintain this new orientation, to reinforce this "new" pattern.

After two sessions, Betty calls me, slightly frantic. "I just got out of a chair without pain for the first time in three years! Is that even possible?"

Indeed, it is.

Another example is Ann, who called recently for an exercise orientation. When she arrived, I recognized her: She had come in two years earlier, had one session, and never came back. She explained that the recumbent bicycle made her arthritic knees hurt, so she stopped—doing anything. In those two years, she had lost weight, specifically muscle weight from disuse and atrophy. She had also lost function, and what little muscular support she had for her arthritic knees had diminished. So her pain had increased. I explained this vicious cycle to her and we talked at length about the pain/fear avoidance model. She got it. She worked through her pain on the machines and is doing just fine now. Better than fine: her strength and function are vastly improved and her pain is now gone.

YOUR PRESCRIPTION:

Don't let pain become permanent:

1. If you feel a new pain or an old one getting worse, take a break. Shake it out.
2. Try again, paying attention. If the pain increases, stop. Take the day off. Then try again.
3. If the pain returns, don't wait. Find a specialist who can help you identify the cause and work through it.

CHAPTER 4: You Are Smarter Than Your Fitbit

I am now going to add you to an exercise experiment—with one caveat. For the purpose of this experiment, everyone is 50 years old. If you are younger, I am sorry, you are now 50 years old. If you are older—and far too wise to participate in such trivial nonsense—then I am sorry, you are now 50 years old.

The first person in your group is 5'4" and weighs 200 pounds. She has a high fat mass, a low muscle mass and a limited history of exercise.

The second person is 5'10" and weighs 160 pounds. He has low fat mass and low muscle mass. He has asthma from smoking and has survived one heart attack.

The third person is 6' and weighs 165 pounds. She has low fat mass and high muscle mass. She is a world champion masters rower.

The fourth person is you. You are X tall and weigh X pounds. You have X fat mass and X muscle mass. Your exercise and dietary habits are X. And you are 50 years old. Again, sorry.

For this experiment, all four of you will go see your physician for an exercise prescription. Granted, you don't have the same physician, and that's OK because, since 1970, doctors have generally been following the same guidelines for cardiovascular health. Your physician points toward an exercise poster on his wall that shows a heart rate intensity graph based on your age. He shows you on the graph that your heart rate, during exercise, should be 119 beats per minute, representing 70% of 220 minus your age. Based on the work of doctors Fox and Haskell circa 1970, this is gospel—and this gospel is embedded in the electronics of countless gym machines that will squawk at you if you don't follow it.

But you tell me, based on yourself and the other three people in this experiment, does this make any sense? I think not, and I hope that you think not. A few years ago I implemented a post cardiac rehab program with a nearby hospital and every patient was given an expensive heart rate monitor, so we had the opportunity to test the 220 minus age formula. It did not work—at all. It was too hard for most, too easy for some, and for others on medications like beta blockers it was simply impossible.

We now know that hearts, like people, come in different shapes and sizes. Some hearts perform optimally at very high rates and some at comparatively low rates. One type of heart isn't better than the other. It is simply that they are different. So we got rid of the heart rate monitors.

What do we do? Well, the answer is wonderfully simple, and it's called RPE, Rate of Perceived Exertion. It's a scale from one to ten. One is breathing. Ten is barely being able to catch your breath. One is sitting on the couch eating Cheetos. Ten is sprinting up a hill with the couch on your back and the Cheetos cheetah on the couch snarling at you. You get to create your own metaphor, your own one to ten. That's part of what makes it so brilliant. The other part is that the scale automatically adjusts to your body and your physical condition from one moment to the next.

Now here is the equation for basic aerobic exercise: Your effort level should be 3–4 out of your 10. Not 5, not 6, not the intensity of the guy working out next to you because your ego is threatened, not 9 because the girl next to you is inadvertently threatening your masculinity, and not necessarily the same pace that your 3–4 was yesterday. It's 3–4, right this moment.

This 3 to 4 pace may seem too easy to some, and it is somewhat counterintuitive to our "more/harder/better" culture, but less stress actually leads to more adaptation and improved fitness. Adaptation trumps stress, and this has been proved, time and time again, even at the Olympic level.

So if you want to train effectively and at the right intensity, dial in to a conversational pace of 3–4 out of 10, and know that you are training smarter, at a seemingly lower intensity, while achieving better results. Sing a few lines of a favorite tune while you exercise. If you can't, you're working too hard.

YOUR PRESCRIPTION:

In addition to lower intensity aerobic training, add some HIIT work! HIIT stands for "high-intensity interval training." Let's say your basic exercise is on a stationary bike or is a walk in the park. After about 10 minutes at your RPE of 3–4, increase your pace for 15 seconds to an RPE of 5–6. Then return to your RPE 3–4 pace for 45 seconds. Repeat that for a total of three to five sets. Congratulations! You have just completed a High Intensity Interval Training session with a work/rest ration of 1:3.

You can manipulate a HIIT session by fiddling with three variables: the volume of work, the ratio of work to rest, and the intensity of the work. If you are exercising aerobically five days a week, add one or two HIIT sessions per week at an RPE of 5, maybe Tuesday and Friday. After a couple of weeks at 15 seconds on/45 seconds off, increase to 30 seconds on/90 seconds off. You have now changed the volume of work while maintaining the same work/rest ratio of 1:3. After a couple more weeks, switch to 30 on and 60 off. Now you have changed the work/rest ratio to 1:2. Next try the same thing at an RPE of 6, changing the intensity. Books have been written on the best formulas, but you don't need them. Just tune in to your own body and play.

And remember to ditch the dated heart rate stuff and find your own 3-4 range. When you can sing me your favorite song while exercising, you know you're there.

CHAPTER 5: We Are All Athletes

Essentially, I train a seventy-year-old hip replacement patient the same way I train an elite athlete. Sure, the loads and speeds are different, but the principles are the same. We are *all* athletes—just training for different activities.

Rowing is an activity.

Getting off the toilet seat is an activity too.

The basic idea for any movement is this; identify the weakness in the neuromuscular pattern, retrain the pattern until it is ingrained in the brain and the muscle, then strengthen the pattern. Seems simple and logical enough, but too often the first two steps are either ignored or simply not known.

Having your body in alignment is essential for allowing your muscles to do their job. Malalignment inhibits muscle function. A perfect example is valgus collapse of the knee (knock-kneed). If your knee caves in toward your midline the reason could be a host of contributing factors: pronation of the foot, tight IT (iliotibial) band, muscle atrophy, or weakness and pain, to just name the most common. Once the contributing factors are identified, they can be corrected, loosened, strengthened, and visually and physically manipulated.

Visually manipulated means this; if you are on your trusty recumbent bike and your knee is caving in as you pedal, you need to visually will your knee to track over your foot where it belongs! This is part of the neuromuscular reeducation process, and I'll talk more about it in the next chapter. The same is true for all activities, such as getting out of a chair or climbing stairs. Because you lack the kinesthetic awareness to know that your knee is out of whack, you need to look down at it and see it before you can know to make a correction. Without this initial and vital component, every step, every pedal, and every repetition you perform will be reinforcing the *wrong pattern*. One of the things a professional athlete knows is the importance of reinforcing the right pattern.

Once the correct patterning is firmly ingrained, then we can focus on strengthening the pattern. That's the fun part. As the New Guinea proverb says, *Knowledge is only a rumor until it is in the muscle.*

YOUR PRESCRIPTION:

Be a daily athlete. We are all athletes, and our field of play is the real world: So our training had better include strength training, because we do it every day. Don't think so? Let's take a look:

Getting out of bed, getting off the toilet, getting off of your chair, and getting in and out of your car are variations of the ubiquitous *squat.*

Lifting your kids or grandkids, hoisting a laundry basket, and lifting groceries out of your car are just three forms of *dead lift.*

Now let's combine upper and lower extremity movements (which require tremendous core support). For example, you are sitting in a chair holding an infant under her armpits, facing each other. You stand up and press her overhead. She screams with delight. You have just performed a *squat-press* and are a functional rock star.

Later in the day, you lift a box of tax receipts and place it in an overhead cabinet. That is a *clean and press* and now you are an Olympic functional rock star.

If you cannot perform any of these movements without some form of assistance, including "cheating" with momentum, you are losing functional strength and should be taking measures to combat that loss.

CHAPTER 6: This is Your Brain on Exercise

In the mid-1990s, while still a fairly young Post Rehabilitation Conditioning Specialist, I opened my first facility in the San Francisco Bay Area devoted to orthopedically sound exercise protocols, specifically for hip and knee replacement patients. I had been a trainer for about 10 years prior to that, and what I had found in running other gyms was a serious lack of expertise in the field of exercise as medicine—as protocoled treatment for specific medical conditions.

So, armed with my newly earned moniker and its associated skill set, I set up shop and started implementing post-rehab programs for all things orthopedic. Being new to a new field—a field viewed with some skepticism by the medical community and patients alike—I was vigilant about not straying outside of the established protocols. So I documented every movement within every session, and dotted every "I" and crossed every "t" in my Physician and Physical Therapy progress reports. Basically, I was trying not to step on anyone's toes.

The thing I learned, seeing an average of 12 clients a day, year after year, is that a lot of our success stories—the physical and mental improvements I documented every day—flew in the face of much of the current medical dogma of the time. We didn't step on toes. We stomped on them.

Rheumatoid arthritis: "No exercise: pharmacological intervention only." [Wrong]

Osteoarthritis pain: "No exercise: bed rest." [Wrong.]

Cancer: "No exercise: Need to conserve energy for treatment." [Wrong.]

Lymphoma: "Don't lift anything heavier than your purse." [Wrong.]

Cognitive decline, Alzheimer's, Parkinson's, stroke: "Well, you are born with a finite number of brain cells that will only decrease as you age, so not much you can do there." [Wrong. Wrong. Wrong. Wrong.]

Today, we know that exercise is good for rheumatoid arthritis, osteoarthritis, cancer, lymphoma, and pretty much everything else. But the most important realization is about neuro-plasticity, the ability of the brain to morph in response to stimuli, and neurogenesis, the regeneration of brain cells. Before the 1990s, and people like Swedish neuroscientist Peter Eriksson, the medical community did not recognize those concepts to be even plausible.

Now we know that exercise is the best way to:

Grow new neurons in the brain;

Integrate them into neural networks;

Increase cognitive function and decrease cognitive decline; and

Improve insulin sensitivity and decrease inflammation
in brain tissue.

With exercise, you train your body to train your brain to train your body to... you get the idea. So how do you train even smarter?

Keep in mind that all human movement is a pattern. Getting out of a chair is a pattern of connected movements. So is making a cup of coffee, putting on your pants, and brushing your teeth. When we do something over and over again the same way, we are reinforcing a neuromuscular pattern. The upside to reinforcing a neuromuscular pattern, such as a baseball player taking 500 swings a day, is that we get really good at it. The downside is that we don't get good at anything else. We adapt and stagnate. If our environment throws us a curveball, we may not be prepared to react—and that can mean injury. Even if we don't get injured, we're not forcing our brain to refresh itself with new neural networks. Fortunately, new networks can be as simple as a single change of step.

The neuroscience of exercise is analogous to the neuroscience of vacations. If we go to the same place every year, our vacations seem shorter—and refreshment diminishes—because our experiences are not different enough to create distinct memories. Twenty years of vacations fade into one blurred memory, and the twenty-first year feels almost over almost before it begins. By the same token, grinding out the miles on a treadmill, year after year, while probably better than nothing, is not nearly so good as learning to salsa, to box, and to swing on a trapeze.

Patterns are good—as long as you are continually making new ones. Let's say you have walked to the train every day for 20 years on your way to work. For 20 years, as you approached the stairs to ascend to the terminal platform, you have taken the first step with your right foot. So that pattern is firmly cemented in your neuromuscular memory. But tomorrow, you're going to take that first step with your left foot, and by doing so you will open a new conversation between your brain and your body. You will start a fantastic neuromuscular dialogue where, in this instance, your muscles will make your brain a bit smarter and, should you choose to continue to lead with your left foot, your brain will reciprocate and make your muscles smarter! That is the conversation we all need to have—and keep having. You might want to skip to work. You might want to skip work and go row a boat.

So what is the secret ingredient known to grow new neurons in the brain, integrate them into the neural network, increase cognitive function and decrease cognitive decline, while at the same time improving insulin sensitivity and decreasing inflammation in the brain tissue? I'll give you a hint. Actually, I'll give you the answer: It's exercise.

The *Journal of the American Medical Association* recently published a study of "elderly" individuals who exercised, on average, 20 minutes a day for 24 weeks. That group demonstrated a 1,800 percent improvement in memory, language ability, attention, and other cognitive functions as compared to the control group.

The mind/muscle connection is indeed a strong one, and it's never too late to train your brain to train your body to get stronger! More on that next.

YOUR PRESCRIPTION:

Every time you perform an action, correctly or incorrectly, your brain "learns" how to create more efficient neural pathways. Think of an efficient neural pathway as Interstate 5 from Canada to Mexico. A straight shot. Think of an inefficient neural pathway as the 101/405 interchange in Los Angeles—from southern California to the depths of hell with delays and a potential for overheating; not so straight of a shot. The more you practice a movement (pattern) the smoother it gets as your brain and muscles integrate and innervate. The more you introduce and practice foreign patterns, the more stimulated— and ultimately smarter—your brain and muscles will become! Here are two examples—give them a go:

1. Brush your teeth with your non-dominant hand. You are now stuck in LA traffic without a map and have created a toothpaste-based Jackson Pollack all over your bathroom vanity.

2. The next time you approach a set of stairs, lead with your non-dominant foot as opposed to your dominant foot. Take note of how that feels and how your body responds. It will adapt, your body will get "smarter," and the world will be a happier and more interesting place!

CHAPTER 7: You Can Get Stronger

I started training Michelle in 2005. An accomplished violinist and deputy district attorney, she had the drive and intelligence that I thought would parlay deftly into the practice of rowing. And they did. Michelle became an athlete. She had no athletic background, yet at 53 years of age she immersed herself in what is arguably the most physically demanding of all sports.

An ergometer is a rowing machine that measures power. It is a cold, unflinching, uncaring machine. Every February rowers from all over the world flock to Boston and other satellite sites to row 2,000 meters as fast and as hard as they can on the "erg." While a small percentage of the elites are out to break world records or get noticed by national teams, most are testing their own personal limits, seeing how they stack up in their age category, trying to hit their own personal bests, etc. While the numbers may be different for each person, the commitment to the training and the willingness to endure the pain of an erg test is no less real for a fifty-something professional woman than it is for an Olympian—maybe even more so.

Two years ago, after Michelle's right arm stopped working during a training row, she was diagnosed with brain cancer. Today, two years after brain surgery, chemo, ongoing therapy, training, and adapting to a new life, Michelle has bested her 2,000-meter erg score by exactly two seconds in preparation for the February contest.

Michelle is my answer to anyone who says that they can't: can't get better, stronger, fitter. You *can*.

When Forgetfulness is a Big Fat Win

When Llyssa came to us one April, she hobbled in with a cane. The cane had become an essential limb upon which she was dependent. That first day, I put Llyssa on a recumbent stepper. My intention was to set the resistance at 1.0, the lowest possible resistance, and start her off with simple "range of motion" work. The minimum wattage to turn on the monitor is in the four to seven watt range. The problem? Llyssa did not have the strength to produce four watts of power. She couldn't even get the monitor to turn on. We resorted to the trusty stopwatch. I decided that if I could at least get Llyssa to move her legs back and forth for one minute, two minutes, three minutes, we would call that a win and call it a day.

And so the days began, and the minutes increased. And then the monitor turned on. Eureka! Llyssa had produced four watts of power. Then she produced five, then seven, ten, 11, 15, 20, all the way to 31 watts of power. So we increased the time to ten minutes on the recumbent stepper, then added more machines: an upper body ergometer, a rowing ergometer, a recumbent elliptical, and a ski simulator.

Last week as I sat at my desk, I looked up to see Llyssa smiling—beaming, really. You could feel her happiness and excitement bursting throughout the room as others exercised around her. She was standing, arms outstretched, fists clenched in victory, as she proclaimed, "I forgot my cane!" Members clapped and congratulated her. She had broken free from her seemingly inextricable appendage. Yesterday, Llyssa leg pressed 160 pounds. I don't think she will forget that anytime soon.

And I hope you don't, either. If Michelle can best her pre-cancer rowing time and Llyssa can go from zero to 31 watts of power, the odds are pretty good that you can beat whatever you think is beating you.

YOUR PRESCRIPTION:

Improvements in strength and aerobic fitness are never completely linear; throughout your journey there will be peaks and valleys, successes and setbacks, and that is normal and perfectly OK. In the beginning, the improvements will be noticeable. As you adapt and become more fit, the improvements will be more finite; Again, totally normal. Even maintenance is better than decline!

CHAPTER 8: On Learning to Fly

I feel immense pride and satisfaction in my clients' successes and progressions. They prevail over their personal demons, blast through their plateaus—physical and otherwise, and they break the chains of their seemingly unbreakable, often self-imposed restrictions. The real, whole truth is that there is enlightenment in the physical realm just as there is enlightenment in the philosophical and spiritual realms. In fact I would argue that true enlightenment is the perfect balance of the three. That is my religion, that is what I preach, and that is the topic of this sermon.

As I've discussed in other chapters we all, as athletes, have to process information in a specific order to truly "understand" that information. In this case, the information is physical movement and the application of strength and then power within that movement. The order goes like this; learn the form first (neuromuscular patterning and reinforcement), then learn strength, and then learn power. Once you have truly "learned" the given task inside and out, backwards and forwards, at varying speeds and resistances, then that information is in the body and we can stop thinking about it. We transfer the information from the brain to the muscle.

This is what the athlete does.

Any hiccup along the way is identified and addressed before continuing with the learning process. Not doing so will retard not only the learning process but also the quality of the end application. If we cheat and ignore the hiccups along the way, we only end up cheating ourselves. What holds true in the intellectual world holds true in the physical. Common hiccups during this process might be injury, weakness, fear, pain avoidance, and—probably the most common—*thinking too much*. When you think too much, you get in your own way and your body can't do its job. When you let go, you fly.

Janet is a full-tilt, one-woman brain trust of smarts: keen of intellect, keen of wit, keen of observation. But the downside to all of that cerebral activity is…a lot of cerebral activity. That internal chatter is disruptive for her. We have worked together as trainer and client for one year now, with consistency and clear goals: get aerobically fit, get strong, get powerful, increase energy and confidence, and look good doing it. Her transformation has been remarkable and inspiring, but also fairly textbook because she is consistent and focused. She shows up—which, you will remember, is the first and most important step.

Three days ago, I saw the first signs of the final stage of Janet's transformation. Her muscles were starting to recognize that her brain was getting in the way. Her *brain* had been telling her brain that for some time, but that's not how we learn, is it?

This morning's mighty workout confirmed it. Janet is learning to let go and learning to fly. Janet is an athlete.

YOUR PRESCRIPTION:

When it comes to mastering any movement, one must follow this progression: Pattern before Strength, Strength before Power.

CHAPTER 9: There Are No Excuses

At our gym facilities, which offer medically protocoled exercise programs, the practice of throwing big sticks about haphazardly is frowned upon. Overhead throwing motions with big sticks can be particularly hard on ageing shoulders dealing with adhesive capsulitis, arthritis, bursitis, rotator cuffitis (ok I made that word up) and impingement syndrome, to name a few. But if you were to throw a big stick it would probably hit a Barbara or a Bill, alone or in combination. These were popular names of the Boomer generation. Here is a Bill story.

Bill just celebrated his three-year anniversary at *Baxter Fitness Solutions*. When Bill came to me, he had spent the last seven months bedridden in an assisted-care facility.

His children finally said, "Enough's enough. We need to get you moving." Waist belt firmly secured, bed transfer to wheelchair, wheelchair transfer to car, car to gym, car transfer to wheelchair, wheelchair to gym, Bill came to me. "Well, waddya think?" ask his kids.

"I'm game if you are," I say.

They were. Bill's daughter Helen even started working out

right then, and she continues to come in with her dad. Today, tall and handsome and ever-friendly, Bill enters the gym under his own power; no more wheelchair. No more assisted care facility.

In November he will be 92. Man, I love my job.

YOUR PRESCRIPTION:

Everyone's progress is an individual journey, not to be compared or measured against someone else's. Take small "steps" if need be. A little bit at a time with consistency will always beat out too much done at once!

CHAPTER 10: Don't Be a Pain in the Hip

Ida Rolph, the Yogi Berra of myofascial structural integration therapists, says, "It is where it ain't." What she means is that where you feel your pain can often be a symptomatic referral originating in a different anatomical address altogether. Yes that was triple-A alliteration, and I'm just getting warmed up, and THAT was two baseball jargon references for Mr. Berra. Stay with me kids, I move quick….

Hip pain is sneaky like that. As I mentioned before, hip pain generally presents one of three ways: in the front, on the side, or in the back—specifically the medial glute area. If you have hip pain, knowing where it presents tells you a lot about the root cause of that pain and how to treat it. Hip pain that presents from the backside is typically muscular in origin and can impact the sciatic nerve. We will pass on that for today. Hip pain that presents in the front is what we call "true" hip pain, and here you probably want to see a doc and get an x-ray. We are definitely passing on that for today. But hip pain that presents on the side is a hobbled hipped horse of a different color (yes, that was a shameless triple-H alliteration, and if there was such a thing as a triple-H ball club, I would be *the* Yogi Berra of Medical

Exercise Specialist authors, but alas...).

The iliotibial band is an incredibly thick, strong, stubborn strip of fascia that runs from the hip (iliac crest) and glute area to the kneecap and tibia, hence the name. Tight IT Bands can do terrible things to knees and hips and backs and feet and checkbooks and moods and marital bliss and really ruin your day.

Case in point: mystery lady comes in to our facility with her husband. She has not slept through the night for six weeks, complaining of hip pain that presents on the side. She saw an orthopedic surgeon, who told her she has an impinged nerve in her back and needs surgery. She comes in to the gym with no appointment since she was in the neighborhood having just had her preoperative anesthesiologist meeting because she is going to have surgery on her spine to fix her hip pain. She sits down in a chair as we talk. I sit down on the floor next to her chair as we talk. Based on the information she has given me, I stick my elbow in the side of her leg. Later, the fire department was able to extract her from the ceiling tiles (kidding), and her husband was impressed with the velocity at which she shot out of the chair, but the point was made. Mystery woman had a bad case IT Band Friction Syndrome. I worked on her for five minutes.

Honestly: five minutes.

The next morning she called to report that she had slept through the night—pain free—for the first time in six weeks. She cancelled her surgery.

The cautionary tale here is this; I see that same scenario, or variations on it, maybe a dozen times a month. Even Yogi Berra would agree that *that* is no joke.

Don't get me wrong: sometimes, surgery is the right choice, most notably when pain and loss of function have affected your quality of life. You'll want to make an informed decision.

YOUR PRESCRIPTION:

Consider different disciplines for musculoskeletal diagnosis and treatment, such as physical therapy, chiropractic, physiatry, massage therapy or a combination of these. You could not only cancel the pain but also the surgery appointment.

CHAPTER 11: A Word to the Wise

OK, soap box time: the top ten most expensive medical issues cost the United States $591,800,000,000 per year. That's five hundred ninety one billion, eight hundred million dollars. US dollars. Per year. That is 17.9 % of the Gross Domestic Product. That list, from one to ten, is as follows:

#1 Heart disease

#2 Trauma

#3 Cancer

#4 Mental illnesses

#5 Osteoarthritis

#6 Chronic obstructive pulmonary disease

#7 Hypertension

#8 Diabetes

#9 Hyperlipidemia

#10 Back problems

Since 1975 health care expenditures have exceeded the GDP by, on average, 2.1% annually.

Granting that two-thirds of cancers are caused by unhealthy lifestyle choices, and granting that 85% of COPD is caused by smoking, that still leaves eight of the ten issues listed above directly treatable through EXERCISE. The two exceptions are mental illness and trauma, although indirectly I would argue that exercise is very good for your mental health as well as your physical health and that a mentally and physically fit person is significantly better prepared to prevent and avoid automobile collisions.

If I'm anywhere near right about this, we can reduce our country's medical costs by $375,150,000,000 per year. That's three hundred seventy five billion, one hundred fifty million dollars. US dollars. Per year. Through EXERCISE. I'm pretty sure that is worth more than a pound of cure, don't you?

Don't thank me now, go out and do something about it—for yourself and for your country. This is your call to arms—stronger, healthier arms!

YOUR PRESCRIPTION:

When you make decisions about your fitness, make sure they are informed decisions. Make sure you do your own research. And when you come across new research, check to see who paid for it! And by all means, stay fit so that you don't add to those health care numbers.

CHAPTER 12: There Is No Magic Pill

Two weeks before the 2012 Olympic Games, I traveled to Hong Kong, where I was honored to serve as consultant and collaborator with hospital therapy clinics throughout the territories as well as the Hong Kong Sport Institute. In addition I managed to squeeze in a book talk at the Royal Hong Kong Yacht Club. That was pretty much the ultimate Andy Baxter trifecta: medical exercise application, elite athletics, and a literary engagement related to rowing. I didn't think it could get any better.

There was a YMCA across the street from the Kowloon Hotel where I was staying. "Perfect," I thought. I could get a workout in before breakfast and start my day off right. I also figured I would run into others of like mind and intent at the gym. I crossed the street, climbed the stairs, signed in, grabbed my towel, and headed to the weight room.

The place was alive with activity. Men and women were working side by side, slogging diligently through their respective routines. The room was full of chatting and laughter—a jocular mix of English and Cantonese (mostly Cantonese). Spectacularly bad Chinese knock-offs of mediocre, 90s-era American pop songs played on the sound system. But what was even *more* glaring than the spectacularly bad knock-offs was that I was the youngest guy in the room! Every single person there was in their 60s, 70s, and beyond.

My trip had just gotten even better.

Later, I asked my friend Yoko about this phenomenon. She answered in a matter-of-fact, casual tone, "Young people just want to work and go clubbing at night. Older people understand the value of exercise."

And they know something about showing up. They know that there is no magic pill but instead the daily ritual of signing in, grabbing your towel, and hitting the machines.

YOUR PRESCRIPTION:

Don't hold your breath that some pharmaceutical company is going to concoct a pretty little pill that will tone your muscles, keep you slim, or otherwise magically keep you healthy. YOU keep you healthy. If you need accountability, create your own fitness log. "Sign in" every day for a month. Write down what you did and for how long. By the end of the month, you will feel better. No magic, just action.

CHAPTER 13: Life Is a Power Endurance Sport

Most athletic endeavors fall to one side of the fitness fence or the other; they are either more anaerobic/power based or they are more aerobic/endurance based. It's not really about being exclusively one or the other, since all energy systems are integrated, but let's just say that a defensive tackle's explosive power is not going to win him any marathons.

Rowing, however, is one of the sublime sports that fit both endeavors. Rowing is a power endurance sport, combining both strength and aerobic capacity with equal, punishing demand.

Every day, I see people battling uncontrollable circumstances, overcoming seeming limitations, "winning" at ageing, and empowering themselves through exercise. Rowing is a metaphor for balanced fitness. My proposition to you: you with arthritis, you with diabetes, you with Parkinson's, you with cancer, you with congestive heart failure, you who are depressed and lethargic—each and every one of you reading this—you are an athlete, and life is a power endurance sport. Find your balance.

Climbing a flight of stairs might be your Everest ascent, and keeping up with your grandkids might be your world cup, but know this; your functional independence and quality of life are depending on you to be powerful and to endure.

YOUR PRESCRIPTION:

Take stock in every victory, no matter how small it may seem. Appreciating and savoring these victories is truly empowering, do not discount them!!

CHAPTER 14: You Don't Know Squat/Deadlift!

I was going to start off this chapter by telling you of my latest research projects at High Point University's health, science, and human performance laboratory in North Carolina. Then I thought I would tell you of a continuing medical education conference that I spoke at on the diabetes epidemic. Then I thought I would tell you about yet another client that turned 92 (yay!). But the story that I just heard this morning takes precedent.

Deborah has been with us since 2008. All those years of consistent exercise would qualify her as quite fit (remember: we are all athletes). Yesterday, Deborah was driving her friend—we will call her Betty—to some appointments and to wrap up some loose ends before leaving on a trip. Betty is 76 years old, and her current state of mobility leaves something to be desired. Deborah pulled up to the curb at their destination. As Betty exited the car to the curb, she tripped and fell in a heap. Deborah ran around the car to assess the damage. Betty was OK, but she couldn't get up.

She explored her options: "If I crawl over to that tree, possibly I could pull myself up. Or maybe if we open the car door, I could work my way up from there…." One thing was certain; Betty was not able to get up under her own power.

Deborah looked at Betty, looked at the tree, and looked at the car door. Hmmm. She positioned herself behind Betty, dropped into a sumo squat position, hooking her arms under Betty's, and in one swift, powerful motion, she stood up, taking Betty with her to a full standing position. "There, no problem!"

Betty looked at her in astonishment and said (you can't make this stuff up, folks), "Wow, I need to go to Baxter's!"

Deborah's typical cheery smile and twinkly-eyed sparkle were both even more cheery and sparkly when she told me this.

Deborah is 85. She is proof positive that you can get stronger at any age. The large and powerful quad, glute and hamstring muscles provide excellent support and protection for aging joints as well.

YOUR PRESCRIPTION:

Squats and Dead Lifts may sound like movements only performed among the pantheon of power lifters. In fact these are functional strength movements that we perform in our everyday lives. Learn to do these power moves properly and your potential strength is practically limitless!

CHAPTER 15: Serious as a Heart Attack

As I write this, eight people are working out in the gym. Three of those eight people are 93 years old—or will be in the next month. That's 37.5% of the present exercising population over ninety: awesome.

Exercise need not be hard, nor arduous, nor reviled, nor a punishment. Exercise should be doable, invigorating, rejuvenating, and enjoyable! To ensure that you associate exercise with the latter four adjectives and not the former four adjectives, let's revisit the RPE scale. Remember: RPE stands for Rate of Perceived Exertion, and it's an easy way to gauge your exercise intensity and help prevent over-training and generally beating yourself up—both physically and emotionally. The RPE scale applies specifically to aerobic activities, such as jogging, vigorous walking, cycling, rowing, etc.

(Mary just walked in. She's 93. That's 44.44 %)

Let's start with a recumbent stationary bicycle as an example. First we identify the variables we have to work with, in this case rate RPM (revolutions per minute), resistance, and duration. Unless you are an experienced cyclist, too high of a spin rate introduces momentum and loss of motor control, so keep your RPM's between 45 and 55. As for duration, we will start simple and cycle for five minutes. Now we have turned two of our three variables into constants, allowing us to focus on the one variable: resistance. Using the RPE scale, your resistance level should be around a three or four on a scale of one to ten. I mentioned the RPE scale in an earlier chapter, but for this go-around, let's say a one is walking down the block to the gym and a ten is sprinting uphill while holding your gym's recumbent stationary bicycle over your head.

(I just spotted Mary for a set of incline dumbbell presses. She's 93, folks. 93!)

Back to your RPE. So your perceived exertion is at a about a three and no higher than a four. Currently this is based on five minutes of exercise at a speed of 50 RPM. If either or both of those variables were to change, then it is likely your resistance would change based on your reassessed Rate of Perceived Exertion.

That is the beauty of the system. The numbers on the machine become irrelevant. What is relevant is that *you* have taken control of your individual exercise program in a palatable, invigorating, rejuvenating, and enjoyable fashion. I know a few 93-year-olds who would agree with me.

YOUR PRESCRIPTION:

Try performing your aerobic activity of choice with your mouth closed. This is a simple and effective way to ensure that you aren't overdoing it. If you have to open your mouth to catch your breath you are working too hard.

CHAPTER 16: Really, Just Show Up

Sam is almost always my last client in the evening before we close. Even if the gym is empty, I would never close up early because I know that Sam might pop in during the last few minutes to get in a quick workout. I enjoy his company and look forward to his visits. This May will be Sam's four-year anniversary with us. He is soft-spoken, thoughtful, and he chooses his words carefully. I mention this because shortly after his heart attack a few years ago, Sam was so weak that speaking required a great deal of effort, and choosing his words carefully was a matter not only of intellect but of necessity.

Often, after his workout, Sam will sit quietly in the waiting room and read a magazine, or we will talk shop until closing time. But tonight he is pensive, walking around the facility, seemingly taking inventory of the exercise machines and his relationship with them. There is an energy about him: a happiness. He taps my desk gently and looks around the room. "You know this…this is the best thing I've ever done in my life. I wish I'd started earlier. Hell, I didn't think I'd even be alive this long."

It's never too late. I can recount hundreds of similar stories of people in all states of disrepair who have turned their lives around through the transformative power of exercise. No one person's battle is greater than another's; they are all relative—as are their successes. The foundation to your success, much like the rest of life, is showing up. Yes, that's a theme. Showing up is no small thing.

When the Going Gets Tough

Here's another "just show up" scenario. On Friday, December 6th 2014, a big snowstorm descended upon Ashland Oregon, leaving a half foot of white stuff on the ground. Usually that is no big deal. Maybe the schools call in a snow day and the kids have the day off, but all in all, a bit of snow is still business as usual. Not so this go 'round. The unique contributing differentiator this time was prolonged freezing temperatures. The beautiful, wintry, festive Friday fluff had turned to ice. By Saturday, everything froze. Parking lots turned into ice skating rinks. Streets were simply treacherous. Banks closed. Pipes burst. Schools shut down for a week. Our little town was paralyzed. Two weeks later, there was *still* ice on the sidewalks.

As expected, business suffered. Town activity slowed to a

standstill. When prioritizing the essentials during this unprecedented cold snap, one would assume that making a onetime trip out for bottled water, batteries and canned soup would trump getting a workout, right? The basic necessities of life would certainly triumph over frivolous modalities of vanity, yes? Not as much as you might think when we examine more closely what might be considered frivolous and what is understood as a necessity.

I anticipated that my *older* clientele (my clients are fifty and over, so "older" is 70 and above) would stay home, huddled around their woodstoves eating their canned soup, helpless and shivering, while their younger, more energetic counterparts would be the ones to brave the elements for exercise. I could not have been more wrong.

I took an age inventory of the morning exercisers who showed up, with exacting consistency, during those two weeks. This is a sampling of their ages: 81, 88, 92, 87, 77, 93, 92, 82, 76, and 81. The average age of those ten people is 84.9 years young. Why aren't they at home clinging to their batteries and canned soup? Because their functional independence *depends on their strength and mobility.* That is part of their everyday reality—a necessity—and no one else is going to do that for them. For this group, exercise is neither frivolous nor vain; it is a way of life.

YOUR PRESCRIPTION:

Health and fitness is not seasonal, nor is it vanity based. Health and fitness is essential to your functional, emotional, and spiritual quality of life!

CHAPTER 17: Economies Of Scale

Over dinner last night, my son informed me that one of his teachers had a condition that attacked her "humane system." I told him I suffered from the same condition and now I hate puppies and small children.... (☺)

Scales are evil. Maybe not as evil as tyranny or prejudice or reality TV, but not far behind. I hate scales. The scale, much like other elements in the world of health and fitness, gives you one piece of information without disclosing other relevant pieces of information. The scale does not paint a complete picture, and this fact becomes ever more hazardous as we age.

Muscle is metabolically active tissue. Fat is not. We are losing, on average, four-tenths of one pound of muscle per year after the age of 50 through the process of Sarcopenia. So if a 65-year-old steps on the scale and sees that she has lost six pounds, she might think that is a good thing. But it may not be a good thing. It may be that she has lost valuable muscle mass, which has lowered her metabolic rate and decreased her functional strength. Some of her weight loss will also be water weight, which will have a negative impact on brain and muscle function.

Here is a real-world example of healthy weight loss. A client of mine, let's call her Irene, went in for a checkup after six months at our facility. She had lost four pounds. At least that is what the scale said. But remember that the scale is giving you a skewed, one-dimensional slice of reality without the substance to give it any meaning whatsoever, like the *Jersey Shore*. What a body composition analysis would show was that Irene's four-pound net weight loss was actually a twelve-pound fat mass loss and an eight-pound muscle mass gain while dropping multiple pant sizes along the way.

And then the Belly Fat

Not only is the scale a skewed and limited assessor of health, so is the average person's understanding of fat.

In my daily interactions with all manner of folk in multiple exercise facilities, I probably see, on average, fifty people per day. That's fifty people per day, five days a week. That's 250 people a week, 1000 per month. You get the idea. So, over the last fifteen years of working specifically with people from the age of 50 to 99 years old, roughly 180,000 of you have asked me a question, directly or in a fantastically round-a-bout way, pertaining to belly fat.

You ask, "How do I strengthen my core?"

I say, "You mean 'how do I get rid of belly fat?'"

Than you say, either sheepishly or just plain relieved that I called it for what it was, "yes."

Or you say, "What types of crunches are best?"

I say, "You mean 'how do I get rid of belly fat?'"

And you say "precisely!" because that wasn't so painful.

Or you say, "Looks like it might rain today" and I say, "You mean 'how do I get rid of belly fat?'"

And you don't say anything because you are marveling at my intuitive power to translate the subtext of what you just said— I know, it's a gift.

Well, for those of you *not* among the 180,000 who have asked or thought of asking that question, here's the answer....

First some basics. Muscle is muscle, fat is fat. Muscle is not fat, nor can it turn in to fat. Fat is not muscle, nor can it turn into muscle. There is no spot reduction. You cannot target fat in a specific area directly by working the muscles in that same area. There is no miracle cream, no magic pill, and no effective *Super Twisty Ab Thingy* as seen on TV for just four monthly payments of $39.95.

What there *is* is a multi-billion-dollar industry feeding on insecurity and perpetuated misinformation. There is that.

Point #1: The "magic pill" is not magic; it is a combination of nutrition and activity. It is caloric intake versus exercise and non-exercise activity thermogenics (Our body's ability to create heat and burn calories).

Point #2: Individual thermogenic properties can vary dramatically from one individual to another, even if two people appear to be the same size and shape.

Point #3: Different muscles have different innervation ratios. How an innervation ratio works: The greater the innervation ratio, the "smarter" the muscle and the more sensitive it is to a given stimulus. Lower innervation ratio muscles are referred to as "dumb" muscles. They are that way out of necessity as they are often bombarded with low intensity, continuous activities. The muscles of the abdomen, calves, and forearms could be considered dumb muscles.

Point #4: Stomach crunches may be only slightly more effective at shedding belly fat than sitting on your couch eating Cheetos while watching infomercials for *Super Twisty Ab Thingies*.

You want to be at a healthy weight and get rid of belly fat? Exercise. Build muscle mass. Skip the Cheetos.

YOUR PRESCRIPTION:

Remember: Your scale is not telling you the whole truth.

CHAPTER 18: The Most Dangerous Word in Exercise

A Hall of Fame NFL running back I knew once suffered a knee sprain. His trainers, some of the best in the world, set up a training protocol that involved aggressive strengthening for the quadriceps muscle, coupled with increasing the flexibility of the hamstring muscle. The result: The quadriceps remained tight and explosively powerful, but the hamstring was comparatively flexible. Weeks later he was back on the field for the first game since his injury. There was considerable buzz and anticipation: How would he perform? Then, on his first play, on national television, in super slow-mo, he took the ball and exploded out of the backfield, powerful legs churning. No one touched him as he reached peak power and stride. What happened next is that his flexible hamstrings couldn't counteract their opposition, so his knee hyper-extended, tearing his hamstring, and he went down like a sack of bricks. Across America, people cringed in empathetic agony, but hardly anyone got the message. His problem had to do with flexibility: too *much* of it!

Okay, so most of us are not pro football players, yet the point is the same. In fact, it may well be more relevant to many of us. Beyond a certain age, most of us are training for life, more specifically quality of life. That quality of life is measured physically by our functional capacity to do all the stuff we like to do—like taking a hike in the mountains, dancing at weddings, and picking up kids and grandkids and pets. These critical life movements each require a specific functional range of motion for each joint involved. Too little range of motion, and we can't do what we want without straining. Too much range of motion, and we too are likely to go down like a sack of bricks.

This is why I don't like to use the word *flexibility*. The culture of the word implies that more is better, and that is simply not true. A healthy goal is not flexibility but rather joint stability with a sufficient, functional range of motion. It sounds complicated, and is—but also is not.

That brings me to yoga, which I take with at least a grain of Sanskrit.

My job as a medical exercise specialist is to assess people's medical conditions, their co-morbidities, and their contraindications, as they relate to exercise programs. Co-morbidity simply means you have more than one medical thing going on at a time. A contra-indication refers to a movement or activity that would be bad for that condition. Things get especially tricky when you have contraindications *within co-morbidities*, meaning that what might be good for one condition could be disastrous for another.

There are so many yoga poses and medical contraindications that it would take a book address them. But let me put it this way: I get a lot of "rehab" business as a result of yoga. The basic problem is that "progress" tends to mean getting deeper into a pose— increasing "flexibility" by creating an increasingly dubious, if not actually dangerous, range of motion. When instructed to breathe and sink deeper into a pose, the first question to ask your instructor is "Why?" Is there a functional good beyond achieving the pose itself? If you're young, you may not have to pay a price for being overly flexible for many years. If you're older, paying the price can happen fast.

Let's say you join a yoga class because your primary goal is to loosen your psoas muscles and strengthen your core. These are pretty common issues, and you inform your instructor of them before class. You also mention that you have spondylolisthesis. Maybe your instructor doesn't know what that is (an anterior slippage of a vertebra), or does and figures the core and psoas work will ultimately help support the spine, so off you go. The contraindication here is that even the most basic back bend (think "upward dog") for someone with spondylolisthesis creates what is commonly known as "the watermelon seed" effect, exacerbating the anterior slippage of the affected vertebra. You had the best of intentions, but now you are sidelined and injured.

My advice is to let your yoga instructor know your various conditions and ask her if she is comfortable with accommodating you. If her eyes glaze over, move on. There are many, many ways to become and remain functionally fit— and they each have pros and cons. But please consider evaluating every program using a very simple measure: Will this movement be useful for the rest of my life?

YOUR PRESCRIPTION:

Since too much flexibility can potentially lead to joint instability and injury, never force a stretch. Just as with RPE—where you stay at a three or four on a scale of one to ten—when you stretch, be aware of your muscle's resistance and listen to your body.

CHAPTER 19: Competition and Community

Every first weekend in April, I and other rowers from all over the world flock to San Diego to race in the Crew Classic to kick off the spring rowing season. Now in my forties, this is my 19th year doing battle in eight-man shells on Mission Bay. Concurrently, at *Baxter Fitness Solutions for Fifty and Beyond*, we are participating in the World Erg Challenge. (Remember, erg is short for ergometer, an indoor rowing machine.) The members and the employees all compete as a team against other health clubs around the world to row as many meters as possible in a one-month period. There are three challenges per year, and we usually finish in the top five—our best showing to date being second place.

Unlike some gyms, I encourage my employees to work out on company time. I think it sends a positive message and develops a certain *esprit de corp*. George works in our Medford location and consistently puts up big-meter numbers. During one challenge, he rowed just over 300,000 meters. That's about 180 miles!

When I'm not on the water competing with former and current Olympians and National Team guys, I'm doing my damnedest to keep up with George. When he's not working the front desk and greeting members, he can be found on the erg or in the back lifting weights. When he is training seriously, as all serious athletes do during a training cycle, he will come in twice a day, double days as we call them, jumping between aerobic and strength workouts. Some people might think that's excessive. I disagree, and so does he. George says his workouts help him in other facets of his life.

George has an unassuming and easygoing nature: a quick-draw smile and a hand-wave hello, he drives a red sports car and is a bit of a chick magnet…. Like you, I am starting to hate George. But then you hear the stories about how he is always around to help a neighbor, befriend a stranger in need, or that a beautiful blonde wants to move in with him and, like you, I am *really* starting to hate George.

In spite of my jealousy, I succumb to the pleadings of all around me and throw my young buck employee a surprise birthday party at the gym. Members bring in baked goods (rrreaallly good ones), we have coffee and other goodies, and all have a grand time and pleasant memories for days to come.

So what is my point? It's this: we are all athletes in this sport of life, and our performance is relative. We don't need to—nor should we—gauge our performance against others, as that is usually counter productive. Individually, we need to find what works for us and go forward with that. That's what I am trying to do, and that's what George does. George who just turned 90.

Happy ninetieth, George!

On the Gym Community

Diana brings me flowers. Diana is both beautiful and happily married. Yet there they sit at my desk: the latest round of colorful, cultivated magnoliophyta straight from her seemingly boundless, magical garden. This has nothing to do with me, you see. Diana brings flowers to the gym for what it gives all of our members: a sense of warmth and connection. That warmth and connection permeate our facilities here in beautiful Southern Oregon.

Yesterday, I received a postcard from Killarney Lake, Ireland. It was from one of our members. When was the last time, while traveling on another continent, you thought to send a postcard to your *gym?* On Monday I will read it aloud to our early morning exercise group, a seemingly disparate bunch that have created strong and lasting friendships based on one common thread: they come to the gym at the same time. They have created community.

Our community is a startlingly powerful one. All matters of interaction occur here. Books are passed back and forth. Recipes are shared. Letters, theater tickets, and photos are given and received. Bodies are strengthened, minds are strengthened, and the bond of community is strengthened—boundless and magical.

YOUR PRESCRIPTION:

Competition is great…for competitions. For your day-to-day fitness, don't compare yourself with others in an unhealthy way. Keep your own fitness goals in mind as you work toward them.

And community is vital. If you haven't already, build a fitness community. Find a friend to work out with. Create a shared fitness goal with someone and challenge each other to reach it.

CHAPTER 20: It's a Lot Easier to Stay in Shape than it is to Get *Back* in Shape

Christmas Eve day was insanely busy. We had people pouring in from opening until closing…crazy. And wonderful energy. I wonder why that is? These aren't the people who think: "I'm gonna slack, therefore I should get in and crush it, and everything will stabilize."

It is really quite the opposite. Folks, it is not the *quantity* of the work in one exercise session, it's the *quality* and the *consistency* of the work over the long haul. If you don't show up then, well, you won't see the desired results.

Not too long ago, I caught up with a fellow athlete and we were decompressing together. He represented the US National rowing team at the highest level, and we had both raced together in the Olympic trials. He confided in me something that I was oddly comforted to hear.

He said, "When I did nothing for a while and came back to the erg (rowing machine), my performance was terrible." And I will vouch for that, his split was gawdawful. What he found out so painfully is this truth: it is a lot easier to stay in shape than it is to get back in shape.

Transformation does not happen overnight. The take-home message is, regardless of whether you are a grandma with a knee replacement, a fifty-something triathlete or a master's power lifter, *consistency is king!*

As I keep saying, we are all athletes in this game of life and we just have to show up to make it work.

YOUR PRESCRIPTION:

Be consistent…the further you get away from a routine the harder it can be to get back to it. Set times in your calendar for the whole month. Recruit a friend and form an exercise pact. Create a menu of different activities to choose from (weights one day, group walk another, swim the next, etc.) so that you can mix things up and keep your routine fresh and enjoyable.

CHAPTER 21: The Pros of Concentric Power Training: Getting More with Less

Quick lesson; when resistance training, the shortening of a muscle under a load is called the concentric phase. The lengthening of a muscle under a load is called the eccentric phase (pronounced "EEE-sentric"). Think of an arm curl with a dumbbell; the "curling" up of the dumbbell is the concentric phase of the biceps muscle. The lowering of the dumbbell is the eccentric phase of the biceps muscle.

Most functional movements are concentric. Most aerobic activity is concentric; walking, running, cycling, rowing—all concentric. Examples of prominent eccentric movements would be big mogul skiing and walking down stairs, both of which can be hard on knees. While eccentric movements have their own validities and applications, we can learn a thing or two from the Olympic lifting community about concentric strength training:

- An eccentric movement can handle a greater load than its concentric counterpart, so it takes more weight to reach peak power.
- Most muscle soreness and tissue damage occurs, predominantly,

during the eccentric phase.

- While eccentric strength movements do elicit improvements in muscle strength and size, they are location and speed specific. They do not translate to functional concentric application.
- Eccentric fatigue compromises the quality/intensity of the concentric work.
- Concentric strength training has shorter recovery time and less muscle soreness, allowing for higher quality/intensity of work and more training sessions.

Sitting down is pretty easy. It is eccentric so you can handle more load (which is, in this case, you) and gravity is offering you encouragement along the way. Once seated, getting up may be another matter. This move is concentric and gravity is working against the load (yep, still you). Furthermore, any extra fat mass that you are carrying is not contributing to the movement because it is not muscle, so it is also working against you.

So scoot out to the edge of your chair with your feet planted parallel, shoulder width apart. Sit up tall, with your chest up and chin level. Extend your arms out in front of you for counter balance. Tilt forward from your hips, without flexing your spine, until your shoulders are over your ankles. Now tighten your stomach and drive up through your heels to a standing position.

Did you make it? Congratulations, you have just performed a concentric squat. In a traditional squat movement, you would begin from a standing position and lower yourself to chair height before changing direction and coming back up. In that scenario the eccentric phase is storing potential energy, like a spring, in what is known as the Stretch-Shortening Cycle (SSC). As you can see, we are not doing that 'cause in the real world, you won't always be afforded that luxury, and we are all athletes in the real world.

Try another one, again setting yourself up with the above postural cues. Try a third. Rest as much as you like in between repetitions if you need to. Do this every day until you can perform a set of ten repetitions. If you can already do ten repetitions, add weight! Hold a five-pound dumbbell at your chest, or a medicine ball, or a water melon, or a grandkid (make sure they sign a waiver). As you press up off the chair, push your dumbbell up overhead in one single, integrated movement. This is a Squat Press.

So, you have mastered and engrained the pattern/form. Then you have built a base of strength. Now it is time to become powerful. Power, somewhat loosely speaking, is strength x speed. Power has significantly more functional application than stand-alone strength. The idea is to take your form and strength and accelerate them—making them both explosive and powerful. The key to making this type of training effective and safe is, you guessed it, to isolate the concentric phase as much as possible.

Case in Point: The Power Squat Press

Ok, so back at your chair with your dumbbell held at your chest, you are going to build power by accelerating the Squat Press movement during the drive phase. This power is a whole-body affair generating from the ground up: from the heels through the legs, butt, core, back, shoulders, arms, and finger tips through whatever you are holding. The very best way to expend this energy in the concentric phase with no eccentric repercussion is to release whatever you are holding at the end of the movement, kind of like a two handed shot putt. You can practice this with a bean bag, or a medicine ball. Watermelon? Not so much. Dumbbell? Definitely not. Grandkid? Get the waiver notarized.

YOUR PRESCRIPTION:

If you haven't already, stop and do those exercises I just suggested.

CHAPTER 22: Overmedicated. Undereducated.

The American healthcare system, it's generating rivers of money that are flowing into very few pockets, and those are the pockets of the manufacturers of medical devices, the big insurers, the pharmaceutical companies. And the owners of those pockets do not want anything to fundamentally change. —Dr. Andrew Weil

People often think it has to be a new drug or a new laser or something really high tech and expensive to be powerful, and they have a hard time believing that these simple choices that we make in our lives each day can make such a powerful difference.
—Dr. Dean Ornish

If I think about what healthcare could be like, it would have a lot more care in it. It would be a very different system that probably would be less high tech. And more high touch. We have a lot more power over how healthy we are than we are willing to take credit for or willing to take responsibility for. And that's part of what a really great healthcare system would do. It would empower patients.
—Shannon Brownlee

These quotes are lifted from the documentary ***Escape Fire: the fight to save American healthcare***. If you haven't seen it, go see it at **www.escapefiremovie.com**. If you have seen it but have loved ones who haven't seen it then you are doing them a disservice by not making them see it. Get it?

Our healthcare system is profoundly broken; no longer a system of care, but a business of treating symptoms. There's no money in it if you get well. That would be bad for business, wouldn't it? The solution to breaking this practically sinister, dystopian stranglehold lies within us, through knowledge and empowerment. Here is just one example.

Terri has been with me for 17 months. She came to me after I had given a talk on fall prevention at a local theater in September of 2015. She has the all too common list of maladies that fall under the heading of *metabolic syndrome*—hypertension, congestive heart failure, diabetes, fatigue, weakness, joint pain, etc. She also has a low resting heart rate, known as Bradychardia.

Terri asked me if my program could help her. I assured her that it absolutely could. I told her with utmost certainty that if she showed up consistently and followed the program I could guarantee positive, measurable results. She had, after all, just listened to me preach the fitness gospel for 90 minutes. Now I challenged her to put that gospel into practice. And so she did, in earnest.

Terri was committed to the program. She was diligent, consistent, compliant, and devoted. Days turned to weeks, weeks to months, and months to seasons. In September 2016 Terri walked into the gym and made her way to my desk. We both knew it was her one year anniversary and I was beaming with pride as she approached to give me her victorious progress report.

"Andy, your program (I'm trying to remain humble in anticipation of her praise, at the at the same time getting ready to jump up and give her a big hug to congratulate her on her success) is NOT working. My blood panels have shown NO improvement, I'm in PAIN, I'm TIRED all of the time, and I feel WEAK and DEPRESSED."

Oh… shit. What??

Exercise is known to have a positive, even profound impact on metabolic, neurologic, cardiovascular, and musculoskeletal conditions. I've been working with people like Terri for **20 years.** She just devoted a full year to this effort and seemingly has nothing to show for it. How can that be?

I quickly switch to a different tack. "Terri, let's take an

inventory of your medications." Here is what we found.

Terri was on a statin for her cholesterol, Carvedilol for hypertension and congestive heart failure and Pioglitazone for Diabetes. She was taking exactly what her doctor had prescribed. What could possibly have gone wrong? Well, it turns out, a whole hell of a lot.

Statins are used to "control" cholesterol levels to prevent heart disease, and that would make perfect sense if there was any correlation between cholesterol and heart disease. There isn't. This is rhetoric propagated by the pharmaceutical industry to make gobs of money. The side effects of statins are muscle pain and damage, elevated blood sugar, diabetes, weakness, fatigue and depression. It is contraindicated for those with diabetes.

Carvedilol is taken to treat hypertension and congestive heart failure. Side effects include drowsiness, weakness, fatigue, joint pain, and bradychardia. It is contraindicated for people with bradychardia.

Pioglitazone is taken to "treat" diabetes. Its side effects are weight gain and muscle pain. It is contraindicated for people with congestive heart failure.

Wow. I mean WOW…

Terri's medications had failed her, even sabotaged her, at

three distinct levels—treatment, compounding side effects, and contraindications. Despite what Dr. Oz tries to shove down our collective throat, metaphorically and in pill form, there is no cure for diabetes in a pill. Taking statins to control cholesterol to prevent heart disease makes about as much sense as taking the bus to control the orbit of the earth to prevent acne; Simply no correlation. The compound side effects of these three medications were hampering the success of the one treatment that would have made a positive impact on all of these conditions – exercise. In fact, her medications were *preventing* her from getting better! And finally, the contraindications could have been disastrous.

So Terri stopped taking her medications. She switched doctors. She embraced a Paleo style diet and cut out newly identified food allergies. I told her that, while not a physician and certainly not pretending to be one, I supported her decision 100% and would be happy to oversee her exercise program. She rededicated herself to a schedule to come in to the gym and meet with me three times per week and stuck to it. Five months later, her new doctor does a full on happy dance in the examination room.

Terri has shown marked improvement across the board. Her cortisol is now normal. Her insulin is down. Her urinalysis is now normal. Her blood sugar is down. Her body composition is changing for the better; body fat down, muscle mass up, body weight down. And medications? Her new doctor recommends a multivitamin, omega 3's, and a probiotic. Now THAT is powerful medicine.

YOUR PRESCRIPTION:

Are you ready to commit to a safe and smart exercise/nutrition lifestyle? Talk to your Physician about your goals as they relate to your medications. Go through a detailed medication inventory with her to identify potential redundancies, contraindications and dosage adjustments. If she is not in line with your new direction, maybe it's time to find another Doc.

CONCLUSION: "Yo, Adrian!"

I recently returned from Philadelphia, where I was training a hospital therapy staff on the benefits of multi-planar resistance for neuromuscular reeducation. That's a fancy way of saying: "train smart."

I had never been to Philadelphia, and there was one thing that I had to do there. If you also saw the movie *Rocky* when you were young, you know what I'm referring to. Yes, I had to run the "Rocky Steps" at the Philadelphia Museum. So, on a cold and crystal clear Friday morning, I went for a nice jog along the Schuylkill River and made my way to the famous steps, easily bounding them two and three at a time to the top, where I snapped a few photos with my phone. Extremely touristy, yes, and not a monumental bucket list moment per se, but it did put a smile on my face. And my smile was also due to gratitude for the fact that my body still does what I tell it to do with relative ease.

Does your body still do what you ask of it? Is there something that you would like to do that might require some forethought and planning—maybe getting ready for a big trip that involves hiking and carrying, or getting as strong as possible prior to a joint replacement to insure a positive outcome? Whatever your scenario, set goals, create a plan of action, and show up.

Once you reach your goals, maintain them. You never know when you'll get the chance to help a fallen friend, give a grandchild a piggy back ride, or run your version of the "Rocky Steps."

Exercise: for strength, for function, for quality of life, FOR LIFE.

Acknowledgements

Sections of several chapters originally appeared in Retire USA

The following chapters appeared as articles in Spirituality & Health:

"Do Not Go Gentle"

"Breaking the Cycle of Fear"

"You Are Smarter Than Your Fitbit"

"This is Your Brain on Exercise"

"The Most Dangerous Word in Exercise"

Made in the USA
San Bernardino, CA
26 May 2017